In order to have a successful Sleeplessness Self Therapy SST you have to start with two things. First, you must be in good terms with all the people which are emotionally important for you. They are not so numerous. 1? 2? 3? So start with reconciliation, when necessary. Second, you must learn to have a distance to your own self. And then continue day after day during 7 to 14 days (7 days should be enough for sleeplessness shorter than 1 month).

Week One

Day 1

Morning

* Whether you slept well or not, try to get out of bed between 6 and 7 o'clock. Never use an alarm clock. Your mind has a perfect feeling for the actual time, so rely on your mind and it will wake you up.

* Never be in a hurry.

* Repeat STOP (10 times every 30 min)

* Say slowly every hour: sun, flower, seven, path, tee, run, yellow, apple, fish, rain, pen, water, smile, talk, life, sky.

* Repeat slowly every hour: I do not care.

* Small physical excercise (10 min)

* Small breakfast.

* Nice talk (no complaints) 20 min. When nobody to talk with, phone or internet conversation oral or written.

* Walk 15 min.

* Imagine all the time people cannot wait to love you, but you must make the first step- a smile, a nice word or both. Only this! Do not be ashamed!

* Do not be serious with your own self. Be funny all the time or at least most of the time.

***

Afternoon

* Never be in a hurry.

* Repeat STOP (10 times every 30 min.)

* Say slowly every hour: sun, flower, seven, path, tee, run, yellow, apple, fish, rain, pen, water, smile, talk, life, sky.

* Repeat slowly every hour: I do not care.

* Dinner and half an hour break (you can sleep).

* Nice talk (no complaints) 30 min. When nobody to talk with, phone or internet conversation oral or written.

* Walk 15 min.

* Imagine all the time people cannot wait to love you, but you must make the first step- a smile, a nice word or both. Only this! Do not be ashamed!

* Do not be serious with your own self. Be funny all the time or at least most of the time.

***

Evening
- Never be in a hurry.
- Repeat STOP (10 times every 30 min.)
- Say slowly every hour: sun, flower, seven, path, tee, run, yellow, apple, fish, rain, pen, water, smile, talk, life, sky.
- Repeat slowly every hour: I do not care.
- Small supper.
- Nice talk (no complaints) 20 min. When nobody to talk with, phone or internet conversation oral or written.
- Walk 15 min.
- Imagine all the time people cannot wait to love you, but you must make the first step- a smile, a

nice word or both. Only this! Do not be ashamed!
- Do not be serious with your own self. Be funny all the time or at least most of the time.

***

Night

- Go to sleep before midnight (22.00- 24.00)

Before sleep

- Take a shower (warm water) 1 min.
- Small physical excercise 3 min.

In Bed

- ALWAYS ALONE during Sleeplessness Self Therapy.
- Repeat STOP (20 times)
- Say slowly untill you fall asleep: sun, flower, seven, path, tee, run, yellow, apple, fish, rain, pen, water, smile, talk, life, sky.
- Repeat slowly every hour: I do not care.

If you cannot fall asleep

- Say slowly untill you fall asleep: sun, flower, seven, path, tee, run, yellow, apple, fish, rain, pen, water, smile, talk, life, sky.

If above does not help

- Stand up and go to the toilet (when possible with as little light as possible)
- Say slowly untill you fall asleep: sun, flower, seven, path, tee, run, yellow, apple, fish, rain, pen, water, smile, talk, life, sky.

If above does not help

- Say STOP untill you fall asleep

If above does not help

- Go to the kitchen and have a very small snack.
- Back to the bed say slowly untill you fall asleep: sun, flower, seven, path, tee, run, yellow, apple, fish, rain, pen, water, smile, talk, life, sky.

If above does not help

- Say slowly untill morning: sun, flower, seven, path, tee, run, yellow, apple, fish, rain, pen, water, smile, talk, life, sky.

Day 2

Morning

* Whether you slept well or not, try to get out of bed between 6 and 7 o'clock. Never use an alarm clock. Your mind has a perfect feeling for the actual time, so rely on your mind and it will wake you up.

* Never be in a hurry.

* Repeat STOP (10 times every 30 min)

* Say slowly every hour: sun, flower, seven, path, tee, run, yellow, apple, fish, rain, pen, water, smile, talk, life, sky.

* Repeat slowly every hour: I do not care.

* Small physical excercise (10 min)

* Small breakfast.

* Nice talk (no complaints) 20 min. When nobody to talk with, phone or internet conversation oral or written.

* Walk 15 min.

* Imagine all the time people cannot wait to love you, but you must make the first step- a smile, a nice word or both. Only this! Do not be ashamed!

* Do not be serious with your own self. Be funny all the time or at least most of the time.

***

Afternoon

* Never be in a hurry.

* Repeat STOP (10 times every 30 min.)

* Say slowly every hour: sun, flower, seven, path, tee, run, yellow, apple, fish, rain, pen, water, smile, talk, life, sky.

* Repeat slowly every hour: I do not care.

* Dinner and half an hour break (you can sleep).

* Nice talk (no complaints) 30 min. When nobody to talk with, phone or internet conversation oral or written.

* Walk 15 min.

* Imagine all the time people cannot wait to love you, but you must make the first step- a smile, a nice word or both. Only this! Do not be ashamed!

* Do not be serious with your own self. Be funny all the time or at least most of the time.

***

Evening
- Never be in a hurry.
- Repeat STOP (10 times every 30 min.)
- Say slowly every hour: sun, flower, seven, path, tee, run, yellow, apple, fish, rain, pen, water, smile, talk, life, sky.
- Repeat slowly every hour: I do not care.

- Small supper.
- Nice talk (no complaints) 20 min. When nobody to talk with, phone or internet conversation oral or written.
- Walk 15 min.
- Imagine all the time people cannot wait to love you, but you must make the first step- a smile, a nice word or both. Only this! Do not be ashamed!
- Do not be serious with your own self. Be funny all the time or at least most of the time.

***

Night

- Go to sleep before midnight (22.00- 24.00)

Before sleep

- Take a shower (warm water) 1 min.
- Small physical excercise 3 min.

In Bed

*ALWAYS ALONE during Sleeplessness Self Therapy.

*Repeat STOP (20 times)

- Say slowly untill you fall asleep: sun, flower, seven, path, tee, run, yellow, apple, fish, rain, pen, water, smile, talk, life, sky.

- Repeat slowly every hour: I do not care.

If you cannot fall asleep

- Say slowly untill you fall asleep: sun, flower, seven, path, tee, run, yellow, apple, fish, rain, pen, water, smile, talk, life, sky.

If above does not help

- Stand up and go to the toilet (when possible with as little light as possible)
- Say slowly untill you fall asleep: sun, flower, seven, path, tee, run, yellow, apple, fish, rain, pen, water, smile, talk, life, sky.

If above does not help

- Say STOP untill you fall asleep

If above does not help

- Go to the kitchen and have a very small snack.
- Back to the bed say slowly untill you fall asleep: sun, flower, seven, path, tee, run, yellow, apple, fish, rain, pen, water, smile, talk, life, sky.

If above does not help

- Say slowly untill morning: sun, flower, seven, path, tee, run, yellow, apple, fish, rain, pen, water, smile, talk, life, sky.

Day 3

Morning

* Whether you slept well or not, try to get out of bed between 6 and 7 o'clock. Never use an alarm clock. Your mind has a perfect feeling for the actual time, so rely on your mind and it will wake you up.

* Never be in a hurry.

* Repeat STOP (10 times every 30 min)

* Say slowly every hour: sun, flower, seven, path, tee, run, yellow, apple, fish, rain, pen, water, smile, talk, life, sky.

* Repeat slowly every hour: I do not care.

* Small physical excercise (10 min)

* Small breakfast.

* Nice talk (no complaints) 20 min. When nobody to talk with, phone or internet conversation oral or written.

* Walk 15 min.

* Imagine all the time people cannot wait to love you, but you must make the first step- a smile, a nice word or both. Only this! Do not be ashamed!

* Do not be serious with your own self. Be funny all the time or at least most of the time.

***

Afternoon

* Never be in a hurry.

* Repeat STOP (10 times every 30 min.)

* Say slowly every hour: sun, flower, seven, path, tee, run, yellow, apple, fish, rain, pen, water, smile, talk, life, sky.

* Repeat slowly every hour: I do not care.

* Dinner and half an hour break (you can sleep).

* Nice talk (no complaints) 30 min. When nobody to talk with, phone or internet conversation oral or written.

* Walk 15 min.

* Imagine all the time people cannot wait to love you, but you must make the first step- a smile, a nice word or both. Only this! Do not be ashamed!

 * Do not be serious with your own self. Be funny all the time or at least most of the time.

***

Evening
- Never be in a hurry.
- Repeat STOP (10 times every 30 min.)
- Say slowly every hour: sun, flower, seven, path, tee, run, yellow, apple, fish, rain, pen, water, smile, talk, life, sky.
- Repeat slowly every hour: I do not care.
- Small supper.
- Nice talk (no complaints) 20 min. When nobody to talk with, phone or internet conversation oral or written.
- Walk 15 min.
- Imagine all the time people cannot wait to love you, but you must make the first step- a smile, a nice word or both. Only this! Do not be ashamed!
- Do not be serious with your own self. Be funny all the time or at least most of the time.

***

Night
- Go to sleep before midnight (22.00- 24.00)

Before sleep
- Take a shower (warm water) 1 min.

- Small physical excercise 3 min.

In Bed

- ALWAYS ALONE during Sleeplessness Self Therapy.
- Repeat STOP (20 times)
- Say slowly untill you fall asleep: sun, flower, seven, path, tee, run, yellow, apple, fish, rain, pen, water, smile, talk, life, sky.
- Repeat slowly every hour: I do not care.

If you cannot fall asleep

- Say slowly untill you fall asleep: sun, flower, seven, path, tee, run, yellow, apple, fish, rain, pen, water, smile, talk, life, sky.

If above does not help

- Stand up and go to the toilet (when possible with as little light as possible)
- Say slowly untill you fall asleep: sun, flower, seven, path, tee, run, yellow, apple, fish, rain, pen, water, smile, talk, life, sky.

If above does not help

- Say STOP untill you fall asleep

If above does not help

- Go to the kitchen and have a very small snack.

- Back to the bed say slowly untill you fall asleep: sun, flower, seven, path, tee, run, yellow, apple, fish, rain, pen, water, smile, talk, life, sky.

If above does not help

- Say slowly untill morning: sun, flower, seven, path, tee, run, yellow, apple, fish, rain, pen, water, smile, talk, life, sky.

Day 4

Morning

* Whether you slept well or not, try to get out of bed between 6 and 7 o'clock. Never use an alarm clock. Your mind has a perfect feeling for the actual time, so rely on your mind and it will wake you up.

* Never be in a hurry.

* Repeat STOP (10 times every 30 min)

* Say slowly every hour: sun, flower, seven, path, tee, run, yellow, apple, fish, rain, pen, water, smile, talk, life, sky.

* Repeat slowly every hour: I do not care.

* Small physical excercise (10 min)

* Small breakfast.

* Nice talk (no complaints) 20 min. When nobody to talk with, phone or internet conversation oral or written.

* Walk 15 min.

* Imagine all the time people cannot wait to love you, but you must make the first step- a smile, a nice word or both. Only this! Do not be ashamed!

* Do not be serious with your own self. Be funny all the time or at least most of the time.

***

Afternoon

* Never be in a hurry.

* Repeat STOP (10 times every 30 min.)

* Say slowly every hour: sun, flower, seven, path, tee, run, yellow, apple, fish, rain, pen, water, smile, talk, life, sky.

* Repeat slowly every hour: I do not care.

* Dinner and half an hour break (you can sleep).

* Nice talk (no complaints) 30 min. When nobody to talk with, phone or internet conversation oral or written.

* Walk 15 min.

* Imagine all the time people cannot wait to love you, but you must make the first step- a smile, a nice word or both. Only this! Do not be ashamed!

* Do not be serious with your own self. Be funny all the time or at least most of the time.

***

Evening
- Never be in a hurry.
- Repeat STOP (10 times every 30 min.)
- Say slowly every hour: sun, flower, seven, path, tee, run, yellow, apple, fish, rain, pen, water, smile, talk, life, sky.
- Repeat slowly every hour: I do not care.
- Small supper.
- Nice talk (no complaints) 20 min. When nobody to talk with, phone or internet conversation oral or written.
- Walk 15 min.
- Imagine all the time people cannot wait to love you, but you must make the first step- a smile, a

nice word or both. Only this! Do not be ashamed!
- Do not be serious with your own self. Be funny all the time or at least most of the time.

***

Night

- Go to sleep before midnight (22.00- 24.00)

Before sleep

- Take a shower (warm water) 1 min.
- Small physical excercise 3 min.

In Bed

- *ALWAYS ALONE during Sleeplessness Self Therapy.
- Repeat STOP (20 times)
- Say slowly untill you fall asleep: sun, flower, seven, path, tee, run, yellow, apple, fish, rain, pen, water, smile, talk, life, sky.
- Repeat slowly every hour: I do not care.

If you cannot fall asleep

- Say slowly untill you fall asleep: sun, flower, seven, path, tee, run, yellow, apple, fish, rain, pen, water, smile, talk, life, sky.

If above does not help

- Stand up and go to the toilet (when possible with as little light as possible)
- Say slowly untill you fall asleep: sun, flower, seven, path, tee, run, yellow, apple, fish, rain, pen, water, smile, talk, life, sky.

If above does not help

- Say STOP untill you fall asleep

If above does not help

- Go to the kitchen and have a very small snack.
- Back to the bed say slowly untill you fall asleep: sun, flower, seven, path, tee, run, yellow, apple, fish, rain, pen, water, smile, talk, life, sky.

If above does not help

- Say slowly untill morning: sun, flower, seven, path, tee, run, yellow, apple, fish, rain, pen, water, smile, talk, life, sky.

Day 5

Morning

* Whether you slept well or not, try to get out of bed between 6 and 7 o'clock. Never use an alarm clock. Your mind has a perfect feeling for the actual time, so rely on your mind and it will wake you up.

* Never be in a hurry.

* Repeat STOP (10 times every 30 min)

* Say slowly every hour: sun, flower, seven, path, tee, run, yellow, apple, fish, rain, pen, water, smile, talk, life, sky.

* Repeat slowly every hour: I do not care.

* Small physical excercise (10 min)

* Small breakfast.

* Nice talk (no complaints) 20 min. When nobody to talk with, phone or internet conversation oral or written.

* Walk 15 min.

* Imagine all the time people cannot wait to love you, but you must make the first step- a smile, a nice word or both. Only this! Do not be ashamed!

* Do not be serious with your own self. Be funny all the time or at least most of the time.

***

Afternoon

* Never be in a hurry.

* Repeat STOP (10 times every 30 min.)

* Say slowly every hour: sun, flower, seven, path, tee, run, yellow, apple, fish, rain, pen, water, smile, talk, life, sky.

* Repeat slowly every hour: I do not care.

* Dinner and half an hour break (you can sleep).

* Nice talk (no complaints) 30 min. When nobody to talk with, phone or internet conversation oral or written.

* Walk 15 min.

* Imagine all the time people cannot wait to love you, but you must make the first step- a smile, a nice word or both. Only this! Do not be ashamed!

* Do not be serious with your own self. Be funny all the time or at least most of the time.

***

Evening
- Never be in a hurry.
- Repeat STOP (10 times every 30 min.)
- Say slowly every hour: sun, flower, seven, path, tee, run, yellow, apple, fish, rain, pen, water, smile, talk, life, sky.
- Repeat slowly every hour: I do not care.

- Small supper.
- Nice talk (no complaints) 20 min. When nobody to talk with, phone or internet conversation oral or written.
- Walk 15 min.
- Imagine all the time people cannot wait to love you, but you must make the first step- a smile, a nice word or both. Only this! Do not be ashamed!
- Do not be serious with your own self. Be funny all the time or at least most of the time.

***

Night

- Go to sleep before midnight (22.00- 24.00)

Before sleep

- Take a shower (warm water) 1 min.
- Small physical excercise 3 min.

In Bed.

*ALWAYS ALONE during Sleeplessness Self Therapy.

- Repeat STOP (20 times)

- Say slowly untill you fall asleep: sun, flower, seven, path, tee, run, yellow, apple, fish, rain, pen, water, smile, talk, life, sky.
- Repeat slowly every hour: I do not care.

If you cannot fall asleep

- Say slowly untill you fall asleep: sun, flower, seven, path, tee, run, yellow, apple, fish, rain, pen, water, smile, talk, life, sky.

If above does not help

- Stand up and go to the toilet (when possible with as little light as possible)
- Say slowly untill you fall asleep: sun, flower, seven, path, tee, run, yellow, apple, fish, rain, pen, water, smile, talk, life, sky.

If above does not help

- Say STOP untill you fall asleep

If above does not help

- Go to the kitchen and have a very small snack.
- Back to the bed say slowly untill you fall asleep: sun, flower, seven, path, tee, run, yellow, apple, fish, rain, pen, water, smile, talk, life, sky.

If above does not help

- Say slowly untill morning: sun, flower, seven, path, tee, run, yellow, apple, fish, rain, pen, water, smile, talk, life, sky.

Day 6

Morning

* Whether you slept well or not, try to get out of bed between 6 and 7 o'clock. Never use an alarm clock. Your mind has a perfect feeling for the actual time, so rely on your mind and it will wake you up.

* Never be in a hurry.

* Repeat STOP (10 times every 30 min)

* Say slowly every hour: sun, flower, seven, path, tee, run, yellow, apple, fish, rain, pen, water, smile, talk, life, sky.

* Repeat slowly every hour: I do not care.

* Small physical excercise (10 min)

* Small breakfast.

* Nice talk (no complaints) 20 min. When nobody to talk with, phone or internet conversation oral or written.

* Walk 15 min.

* Imagine all the time people cannot wait to love you, but you must make the first step- a smile, a nice word or both. Only this! Do not be ashamed!

* Do not be serious with your own self. Be funny all the time or at least most of the time.

***

Afternoon

* Never be in a hurry.

* Repeat STOP (10 times every 30 min.)

* Say slowly every hour: sun, flower, seven, path, tee, run, yellow, apple, fish, rain, pen, water, smile, talk, life, sky.

* Repeat slowly every hour: I do not care.

* Dinner and half an hour break (you can sleep).

* Nice talk (no complaints) 30 min. When nobody to talk with, phone or internet conversation oral or written.

* Walk 15 min.

* Imagine all the time people cannot wait to love you, but you must make the first step- a smile, a nice word or both. Only this! Do not be ashamed!

* Do not be serious with your own self. Be funny all the time or at least most of the time.

***

Evening
- Never be in a hurry.
- Repeat STOP (10 times every 30 min.)
- Say slowly every hour: sun, flower, seven, path, tee, run, yellow, apple, fish, rain, pen, water, smile, talk, life, sky.
- Repeat slowly every hour: I do not care.
- Small supper.
- Nice talk (no complaints) 20 min. When nobody to talk with, phone or internet conversation oral or written.
- Walk 15 min.
- Imagine all the time people cannot wait to love you, but you must make the first step- a smile, a nice word or both. Only this! Do not be ashamed!
- Do not be serious with your own self. Be funny all the time or at least most of the time.

***

Night
- Go to sleep before midnight (22.00- 24.00)

Before sleep
- Take a shower (warm water) 1 min.
- Small physical excercise 3 min.

In Bed
- *ALWAYS ALONE during Sleeplessness Self Therapy.
- Repeat STOP (20 times)
- Say slowly untill you fall asleep: sun, flower, seven, path, tee, run, yellow, apple, fish, rain, pen, water, smile, talk, life, sky.
- Repeat slowly every hour: I do not care.

If you cannot fall asleep
- Say slowly untill you fall asleep: sun, flower, seven, path, tee, run, yellow, apple, fish, rain, pen, water, smile, talk, life, sky.

If above does not help
- Stand up and go to the toilet (when possible with as little light as possible)
- Say slowly untill you fall asleep: sun, flower, seven, path, tee, run, yellow, apple, fish, rain, pen, water, smile, talk, life, sky.

If above does not help

- Say STOP untill you fall asleep

If above does not help

- Go to the kitchen and have a very small snack.
- Back to the bed say slowly untill you fall asleep: sun, flower, seven, path, tee, run, yellow, apple, fish, rain, pen, water, smile, talk, life, sky.

If above does not help

- Say slowly untill morning: sun, flower, seven, path, tee, run, yellow, apple, fish, rain, pen, water, smile, talk, life, sky.

Day 7

Morning

* Whether you slept well or not, try to get out of bed between 6 and 7 o'clock. Never use an alarm clock. Your mind has a perfect feeling for the actual time, so rely on your mind and it will wake you up.

* Never be in a hurry.

* Repeat STOP (10 times every 30 min)

* Say slowly every hour: sun, flower, seven, path, tee, run, yellow, apple, fish, rain, pen, water, smile, talk, life, sky.

* Repeat slowly every hour: I do not care.

* Small physical excercise (10 min)

* Small breakfast.

* Nice talk (no complaints) 20 min. When nobody to talk with, phone or internet conversation oral or written.

* Walk 15 min.

* Imagine all the time people cannot wait to love you, but you must make the first step- a smile, a nice word or both. Only this! Do not be ashamed!

* Do not be serious with your own self. Be funny all the time or at least most of the time.

***

Afternoon

* Never be in a hurry.

* Repeat STOP (10 times every 30 min.)

* Say slowly every hour: sun, flower, seven, path, tee, run, yellow, apple, fish, rain, pen, water, smile, talk, life, sky.

* Repeat slowly every hour: I do not care.

* Dinner and half an hour break (you can sleep).

* Nice talk (no complaints) 30 min. When nobody to talk with, phone or internet conversation oral or written.

* Walk 15 min.

* Imagine all the time people cannot wait to love you, but you must make the first step- a smile, a nice word or both. Only this! Do not be ashamed!

* Do not be serious with your own self. Be funny all the time or at least most of the time.

***

Evening
- Never be in a hurry.
- Repeat STOP (10 times every 30 min.)
- Say slowly every hour: sun, flower, seven, path, tee, run, yellow, apple, fish, rain, pen, water, smile, talk, life, sky.
- Repeat slowly every hour: I do not care.
- Small supper.

- Nice talk (no complaints) 20 min. When nobody to talk with, phone or internet conversation oral or written.
- Walk 15 min.
- Imagine all the time people cannot wait to love you, but you must make the first step- a smile, a nice word or both. Only this! Do not be ashamed!
- Do not be serious with your own self. Be funny all the time or at least most of the time.

***

Night

- Go to sleep before midnight (22.00- 24.00)

Before sleep

- Take a shower (warm water) 1 min.
- Small physical excercise 3 min.

In Bed

- *ALWAYS ALONE during Sleeplessness Self Therapy.
- Repeat STOP (20 times)
- Say slowly untill you fall asleep: sun, flower, seven, path, tee, run, yellow, apple, fish, rain, pen, water, smile, talk, life, sky.
- Repeat slowly every hour: I do not care.

If you cannot fall asleep

- Say slowly untill you fall asleep: sun, flower, seven, path, tee, run, yellow, apple, fish, rain, pen, water, smile, talk, life, sky.

If above does not help

- Stand up and go to the toilet (when possible with as little light as possible)
- Say slowly untill you fall asleep: sun, flower, seven, path, tee, run, yellow, apple, fish, rain, pen, water, smile, talk, life, sky.

If above does not help

- Say STOP untill you fall asleep

If above does not help

- Go to the kitchen and have a very small snack.
- Back to the bed say slowly untill you fall asleep: sun, flower, seven, path, tee, run, yellow, apple, fish, rain, pen, water, smile, talk, life, sky.

If above does not help

- Say slowly untill morning: sun, flower, seven, path, tee, run, yellow, apple, fish, rain, pen, water, smile, talk, life, sky.

***

Week Two

***

Day 1

Morning

* Whether you slept well or not, try to get out of bed between 6 and 7 o'clock. Never use an alarm clock. Your mind has a perfect feeling for the actual time, so rely on your mind and it will wake you up.

* Never be in a hurry.

* Repeat STOP to stop thinking.

* Say slowly to stop thinking : sun, flower, seven, path, tee, run, yellow, apple, fish, rain, pen, water, smile, talk, life, sky.

* Repeat slowly every hour: I do not care.

* Small physical excercise (20 min)

* Small breakfast.

* Nice talk (no complaints) 30 min. When nobody to talk with, phone or internet conversation oral or written.

* Walk 30 min.

* Imagine all the time people cannot wait to love you, but you must make the first step- a smile, a nice word or both. Only this! Do not be ashamed!

* Do not be serious with your own self. Be funny all the time or at least most of the time.

***

Afternoon

* Never be in a hurry.

* Repeat STOP (10 times every 30 hour)

* Say slowly every hour: sun, flower, seven, path, tee, run, yellow, apple, fish, rain, pen, water, smile, talk, life, sky.

* Repeat slowly every hour: I do not care.

* Dinner and half an hour break (you can sleep).

* Nice talk (no complaints) 30 min. When nobody to talk with, phone or internet conversation oral or written.

* Walk 30 min.

* Imagine all the time people cannot wait to love you, but you must make the first step- a smile, a nice word or both. Only this! Do not be ashamed!

 * Do not be serious with your own self. Be funny all the time or at least most of the time.

***

Evening
- Never be in a hurry.
- Repeat STOP to stop thinking.
- Say slowly to stop thinking: sun, flower, seven, path, tee, run, yellow, apple, fish, rain, pen, water, smile, talk, life, sky.
- Repeat slowly every hour: I do not care.
- Small supper.
- Nice talk (no complaints) 30 min. When nobody to talk with, phone or internet conversation oral or written.
- Walk 30 min.
- Imagine all the time people cannot wait to love you, but you must make the first step- a smile, a nice word or both. Only this! Do not be ashamed!
- Do not be serious with your own self. Be funny all the time or at least most of the time.

***

Night
- Go to sleep before midnight (22.00- 24.00)

Before sleep
- Take a shower (warm water) 1 min.

- Small physical excercise 5 min.

In Bed

- ALWAYS ALONE during Sleeplessness Self Therapy.
- Repeat STOP to stop thinking.
- Say slowly untill you fall asleep: sun, flower, seven, path, tee, run, yellow, apple, fish, rain, pen, water, smile, talk, life, sky.
- Repeat slowly every hour: I do not care.

If you cannot fall asleep

- Say slowly untill you fall asleep: sun, flower, seven, path, tee, run, yellow, apple, fish, rain, pen, water, smile, talk, life, sky.

If above does not help

- Stand up and go to the toilet (when possible with as little light as possible)
- Say slowly untill you fall asleep: sun, flower, seven, path, tee, run, yellow, apple, fish, rain, pen, water, smile, talk, life, sky.

If above does not help

- Say STOP untill you fall asleep

If above does not help

- Go to the kitchen and have a very small snack.

- Back to the bed say slowly untill you fall asleep: sun, flower, seven, path, tee, run, yellow, apple, fish, rain, pen, water, smile, talk, life, sky.

If above does not help

- Say slowly untill morning: sun, flower, seven, path, tee, run, yellow, apple, fish, rain, pen, water, smile, talk, life, sky.

Day 2

Morning

* Whether you slept well or not, try to get out of bed between 6 and 7 o'clock. Never use an alarm clock. Your mind has a perfect feeling for the actual time, so rely on your mind and it will wake you up.

* Never be in a hurry.

* Repeat STOP to stop thinking.

* Say slowly to stop thinking : sun, flower, seven, path, tee, run, yellow, apple, fish, rain, pen, water, smile, talk, life, sky.

* Repeat slowly every hour: I do not care.

* Small physical excercise (20 min)

* Small breakfast.

* Nice talk (no complaints) 30 min. When nobody to talk with, phone or internet conversation oral or written.

* Walk 30 min.

* Imagine all the time people cannot wait to love you, but you must make the first step- a smile, a nice word or both. Only this! Do not be ashamed!

* Do not be serious with your own self. Be funny all the time or at least most of the time.

***

Afternoon

* Never be in a hurry.

* Repeat STOP (10 times every 30 hour)

* Say slowly every hour: sun, flower, seven, path, tee, run, yellow, apple, fish, rain, pen, water, smile, talk, life, sky.

* Repeat slowly every hour: I do not care.

* Dinner and half an hour break (you can sleep).

* Nice talk (no complaints) 30 min. When nobody to talk with, phone or internet conversation oral or written.

* Walk 30 min.

* Imagine all the time people cannot wait to love you, but you must make the first step- a smile, a nice word or both. Only this! Do not be ashamed!

* Do not be serious with your own self. Be funny all the time or at least most of the time.

***

Evening
- Never be in a hurry.
- Repeat STOP to stop thinking.
- Say slowly to stop thinking: sun, flower, seven, path, tee, run, yellow, apple, fish, rain, pen, water, smile, talk, life, sky.
- Repeat slowly every hour: I do not care.
- Small supper.
- Nice talk (no complaints) 30 min. When nobody to talk with, phone or internet conversation oral or written.
- Walk 30 min.
- Imagine all the time people cannot wait to love you, but you must make the first step- a smile, a

- nice word or both. Only this! Do not be ashamed!
- Do not be serious with your own self. Be funny all the time or at least most of the time.

***

Night

- Go to sleep before midnight (22.00- 24.00)

Before sleep

- Take a shower (warm water) 1 min.
- Small physical excercise 5 min.

In Bed

- ALWAYS ALONE during Sleeplessness Self Therapy.
- Repeat STOP to stop thinking.
- Say slowly untill you fall asleep: sun, flower, seven, path, tee, run, yellow, apple, fish, rain, pen, water, smile, talk, life, sky.
- Repeat slowly every hour: I do not care.

If you cannot fall asleep

- Say slowly untill you fall asleep: sun, flower, seven, path, tee, run, yellow, apple, fish, rain, pen, water, smile, talk, life, sky.

If above does not help

- Stand up and go to the toilet (when possible with as little light as possible)
- Say slowly untill you fall asleep: sun, flower, seven, path, tee, run, yellow, apple, fish, rain, pen, water, smile, talk, life, sky.

If above does not help

- Say STOP untill you fall asleep

If above does not help

- Go to the kitchen and have a very small snack.
- Back to the bed say slowly untill you fall asleep: sun, flower, seven, path, tee, run, yellow, apple, fish, rain, pen, water, smile, talk, life, sky.

If above does not help

- Say slowly untill morning: sun, flower, seven, path, tee, run, yellow, apple, fish, rain, pen, water, smile, talk, life, sky.

Day 3

Morning

* Whether you slept well or not, try to get out of bed between 6 and 7 o'clock. Never use an alarm clock. Your mind has a perfect feeling for the actual time, so rely on your mind and it will wake you up.

* Never be in a hurry.

* Repeat STOP to stop thinking.

* Say slowly to stop thinking : sun, flower, seven, path, tee, run, yellow, apple, fish, rain, pen, water, smile, talk, life, sky.

* Repeat slowly every hour: I do not care.

* Small physical excercise (20 min)

* Small breakfast.

* Nice talk (no complaints) 30 min. When nobody to talk with, phone or internet conversation oral or written.

* Walk 30 min.

* Imagine all the time people cannot wait to love you, but you must make the first step- a smile, a nice word or both. Only this! Do not be ashamed!

* Do not be serious with your own self. Be funny all the time or at least most of the time.

***

Afternoon

* Never be in a hurry.

* Repeat STOP (10 times every 30 hour)

* Say slowly every hour: sun, flower, seven, path, tee, run, yellow, apple, fish, rain, pen, water, smile, talk, life, sky.

* Repeat slowly every hour: I do not care.

* Dinner and half an hour break (you can sleep).

* Nice talk (no complaints) 30 min. When nobody to talk with, phone or internet conversation oral or written.

* Walk 30 min.

* Imagine all the time people cannot wait to love you, but you must make the first step- a smile, a nice word or both. Only this! Do not be ashamed!

* Do not be serious with your own self. Be funny all the time or at least most of the time.

***

Evening
- Never be in a hurry.
- Repeat STOP to stop thinking.
- Say slowly to stop thinking: sun, flower, seven, path, tee, run, yellow, apple, fish, rain, pen, water, smile, talk, life, sky.
- Repeat slowly every hour: I do not care.

- Small supper.
- Nice talk (no complaints) 30 min. When nobody to talk with, phone or internet conversation oral or written.
- Walk 30 min.
- Imagine all the time people cannot wait to love you, but you must make the first step- a smile, a nice word or both. Only this! Do not be ashamed!
- Do not be serious with your own self. Be funny all the time or at least most of the time.

***

Night

- Go to sleep before midnight (22.00- 24.00)

Before sleep

- Take a shower (warm water) 1 min.
- Small physical excercise 5 min.

In Bed

- ALWAYS ALONE during Sleeplessness Self Therapy.
- Repeat STOP to stop thinking.
- Say slowly untill you fall asleep: sun, flower, seven, path, tee, run, yellow, apple, fish, rain, pen, water, smile, talk, life, sky.

- Repeat slowly every hour: I do not care.

If you cannot fall asleep

- Say slowly untill you fall asleep: sun, flower, seven, path, tee, run, yellow, apple, fish, rain, pen, water, smile, talk, life, sky.

If above does not help

- Stand up and go to the toilet (when possible with as little light as possible)
- Say slowly untill you fall asleep: sun, flower, seven, path, tee, run, yellow, apple, fish, rain, pen, water, smile, talk, life, sky.

If above does not help

- Say STOP untill you fall asleep

If above does not help

- Go to the kitchen and have a very small snack.
- Back to the bed say slowly untill you fall asleep: sun, flower, seven, path, tee, run, yellow, apple, fish, rain, pen, water, smile, talk, life, sky.

If above does not help

- Say slowly untill morning: sun, flower, seven, path, tee, run, yellow, apple, fish, rain, pen, water, smile, talk, life, sky.

Day 4

Morning

* Whether you slept well or not, try to get out of bed between 6 and 7 o'clock. Never use an alarm clock. Your mind has a perfect feeling for the actual time, so rely on your mind and it will wake you up.

* Never be in a hurry.

* Repeat STOP to stop thinking.

* Say slowly to stop thinking : sun, flower, seven, path, tee, run, yellow, apple, fish, rain, pen, water, smile, talk, life, sky.

* Repeat slowly every hour: I do not care.

* Small physical excercise (20 min)

* Small breakfast.

* Nice talk (no complaints) 30 min. When nobody to talk with, phone or internet conversation oral or written.

* Walk 30 min.

* Imagine all the time people cannot wait to love you, but you must make the first step- a smile, a nice word or both. Only this! Do not be ashamed!

* Do not be serious with your own self. Be funny all the time or at least most of the time.

***

Afternoon

* Never be in a hurry.

* Repeat STOP (10 times every 30 hour)

* Say slowly every hour: sun, flower, seven, path, tee, run, yellow, apple, fish, rain, pen, water, smile, talk, life, sky.

* Repeat slowly every hour: I do not care.

* Dinner and half an hour break (you can sleep).

* Nice talk (no complaints) 30 min. When nobody to talk with, phone or internet conversation oral or written.

* Walk 30 min.

* Imagine all the time people cannot wait to love you, but you must make the first step- a smile, a nice word or both. Only this! Do not be ashamed!

 * Do not be serious with your own self. Be funny all the time or at least most of the time.

Day 4

Morning

* Whether you slept well or not, try to get out of bed between 6 and 7 o'clock. Never use an alarm clock. Your mind has a perfect feeling for the actual time, so rely on your mind and it will wake you up.

* Never be in a hurry.

* Repeat STOP to stop thinking.

* Say slowly to stop thinking : sun, flower, seven, path, tee, run, yellow, apple, fish, rain, pen, water, smile, talk, life, sky.

* Repeat slowly every hour: I do not care.

* Small physical excercise (20 min)

* Small breakfast.

* Nice talk (no complaints) 30 min. When nobody to talk with, phone or internet conversation oral or written.

* Walk 30 min.

* Imagine all the time people cannot wait to love you, but you must make the first step- a smile, a nice word or both. Only this! Do not be ashamed!

* Do not be serious with your own self. Be funny all the time or at least most of the time.

***

Afternoon

* Never be in a hurry.

* Repeat STOP (10 times every 30 hour)

* Say slowly every hour: sun, flower, seven, path, tee, run, yellow, apple, fish, rain, pen, water, smile, talk, life, sky.

* Repeat slowly every hour: I do not care.

* Dinner and half an hour break (you can sleep).

* Nice talk (no complaints) 30 min. When nobody to talk with, phone or internet conversation oral or written.

* Walk 30 min.

* Imagine all the time people cannot wait to love you, but you must make the first step- a smile, a nice word or both. Only this! Do not be ashamed!

 * Do not be serious with your own self. Be funny all the time or at least most of the time.

***

Evening
- Never be in a hurry.
- Repeat STOP to stop thinking.
- Say slowly to stop thinking: sun, flower, seven, path, tee, run, yellow, apple, fish, rain, pen, water, smile, talk, life, sky.
- Repeat slowly every hour: I do not care.
- Small supper.
- Nice talk (no complaints) 30 min. When nobody to talk with, phone or internet conversation oral or written.
- Walk 30 min.
- Imagine all the time people cannot wait to love you, but you must make the first step- a smile, a nice word or both. Only this! Do not be ashamed!
- Do not be serious with your own self. Be funny all the time or at least most of the time.

***

Night
- Go to sleep before midnight (22.00- 24.00)

Before sleep
- Take a shower (warm water) 1 min.

- Small physical excercise 5 min.

In Bed

- ALWAYS ALONE during Sleeplessness Self Therapy.
- Repeat STOP to stop thinking.
- Say slowly untill you fall asleep: sun, flower, seven, path, tee, run, yellow, apple, fish, rain, pen, water, smile, talk, life, sky.
- Repeat slowly every hour: I do not care.

If you cannot fall asleep

- Say slowly untill you fall asleep: sun, flower, seven, path, tee, run, yellow, apple, fish, rain, pen, water, smile, talk, life, sky.

If above does not help

- Stand up and go to the toilet (when possible with as little light as possible)
- Say slowly untill you fall asleep: sun, flower, seven, path, tee, run, yellow, apple, fish, rain, pen, water, smile, talk, life, sky.

If above does not help

- Say STOP untill you fall asleep

If above does not help

- Go to the kitchen and have a very small snack.

- Back to the bed say slowly untill you fall asleep: sun, flower, seven, path, tee, run, yellow, apple, fish, rain, pen, water, smile, talk, life, sky.

If above does not help

- Say slowly untill morning: sun, flower, seven, path, tee, run, yellow, apple, fish, rain, pen, water, smile, talk, life, sky.

Day 5

Morning

* Whether you slept well or not, try to get out of bed between 6 and 7 o'clock. Never use an alarm clock. Your mind has a perfect feeling for the actual time, so rely on your mind and it will wake you up.

* Never be in a hurry.

* Repeat STOP to stop thinking.

* Say slowly to stop thinking : sun, flower, seven, path, tee, run, yellow, apple, fish, rain, pen, water, smile, talk, life, sky.

* Repeat slowly every hour: I do not care.

* Small physical excercise (20 min)

* Small breakfast.

* Nice talk (no complaints) 30 min. When nobody to talk with, phone or internet conversation oral or written.

* Walk 30 min.

* Imagine all the time people cannot wait to love you, but you must make the first step- a smile, a nice word or both. Only this! Do not be ashamed!

* Do not be serious with your own self. Be funny all the time or at least most of the time.

***

Afternoon

* Never be in a hurry.

* Repeat STOP (10 times every 30 hour)

* Say slowly every hour: sun, flower, seven, path, tee, run, yellow, apple, fish, rain, pen, water, smile, talk, life, sky.

* Repeat slowly every hour: I do not care.

* Dinner and half an hour break (you can sleep).

* Nice talk (no complaints) 30 min. When nobody to talk with, phone or internet conversation oral or written.

* Walk 30 min.

* Imagine all the time people cannot wait to love you, but you must make the first step- a smile, a nice word or both. Only this! Do not be ashamed!

* Do not be serious with your own self. Be funny all the time or at least most of the time.

***

Evening
- Never be in a hurry.
- Repeat STOP to stop thinking.
- Say slowly to stop thinking: sun, flower, seven, path, tee, run, yellow, apple, fish, rain, pen, water, smile, talk, life, sky.
- Repeat slowly every hour: I do not care.
- Small supper.
- Nice talk (no complaints) 30 min. When nobody to talk with, phone or internet conversation oral or written.
- Walk 30 min.
- Imagine all the time people cannot wait to love you, but you must make the first step- a smile, a

nice word or both. Only this! Do not be ashamed!

- Do not be serious with your own self. Be funny all the time or at least most of the time.

***

Night

- Go to sleep before midnight (22.00- 24.00)

Before sleep

- Take a shower (warm water) 1 min.
- Small physical excercise 5 min.

In Bed

- ALWAYS ALONE during Sleeplessness Self Therapy.
- Repeat STOP to stop thinking.
- Say slowly untill you fall asleep: sun, flower, seven, path, tee, run, yellow, apple, fish, rain, pen, water, smile, talk, life, sky.
- Repeat slowly every hour: I do not care.

If you cannot fall asleep

- Say slowly untill you fall asleep: sun, flower, seven, path, tee, run, yellow, apple, fish, rain, pen, water, smile, talk, life, sky.

If above does not help

- Stand up and go to the toilet (when possible with as little light as possible)
- Say slowly untill you fall asleep: sun, flower, seven, path, tee, run, yellow, apple, fish, rain, pen, water, smile, talk, life, sky.

If above does not help

- Say STOP untill you fall asleep

If above does not help

- Go to the kitchen and have a very small snack.
- Back to the bed say slowly untill you fall asleep: sun, flower, seven, path, tee, run, yellow, apple, fish, rain, pen, water, smile, talk, life, sky.

If above does not help

- Say slowly untill morning: sun, flower, seven, path, tee, run, yellow, apple, fish, rain, pen, water, smile, talk, life, sky.

Day 6

Morning

* Whether you slept well or not, try to get out of bed between 6 and 7 o'clock. Never use an alarm clock. Your mind has a perfect feeling for the actual time, so rely on your mind and it will wake you up.

* Never be in a hurry.

* Repeat STOP to stop thinking.

* Say slowly to stop thinking : sun, flower, seven, path, tee, run, yellow, apple, fish, rain, pen, water, smile, talk, life, sky.

* Repeat slowly every hour: I do not care.

* Small physical excercise (20 min)

* Small breakfast.

* Nice talk (no complaints) 30 min. When nobody to talk with, phone or internet conversation oral or written.

* Walk 30 min.

* Imagine all the time people cannot wait to love you, but you must make the first step- a smile, a nice word or both. Only this! Do not be ashamed!

* Do not be serious with your own self. Be funny all the time or at least most of the time.

***

Afternoon

* Never be in a hurry.

* Repeat STOP (10 times every 30 hour)

* Say slowly every hour: sun, flower, seven, path, tee, run, yellow, apple, fish, rain, pen, water, smile, talk, life, sky.

* Repeat slowly every hour: I do not care.

* Dinner and half an hour break (you can sleep).

* Nice talk (no complaints) 30 min. When nobody to talk with, phone or internet conversation oral or written.

* Walk 30 min.

* Imagine all the time people cannot wait to love you, but you must make the first step- a smile, a nice word or both. Only this! Do not be ashamed!

* Do not be serious with your own self. Be funny all the time or at least most of the time.

***

Evening
- Never be in a hurry.
- Repeat STOP to stop thinking.
- Say slowly to stop thinking: sun, flower, seven, path, tee, run, yellow, apple, fish, rain, pen, water, smile, talk, life, sky.
- Repeat slowly every hour: I do not care.

- Small supper.
- Nice talk (no complaints) 30 min. When nobody to talk with, phone or internet conversation oral or written.
- Walk 30 min.
- Imagine all the time people cannot wait to love you, but you must make the first step- a smile, a nice word or both. Only this! Do not be ashamed!
- Do not be serious with your own self. Be funny all the time or at least most of the time.

***

Night

- Go to sleep before midnight (22.00- 24.00)

Before sleep

- Take a shower (warm water) 1 min.
- Small physical excercise 5 min.

In Bed

- ALWAYS ALONE during Sleeplessness Self Therapy.
- Repeat STOP to stop thinking.
- Say slowly untill you fall asleep: sun, flower, seven, path, tee, run, yellow, apple, fish, rain, pen, water, smile, talk, life, sky.

- Repeat slowly every hour: I do not care.

If you cannot fall asleep

- Say slowly untill you fall asleep: sun, flower, seven, path, tee, run, yellow, apple, fish, rain, pen, water, smile, talk, life, sky.

If above does not help

- Stand up and go to the toilet (when possible with as little light as possible)
- Say slowly untill you fall asleep: sun, flower, seven, path, tee, run, yellow, apple, fish, rain, pen, water, smile, talk, life, sky.

If above does not help

- Say STOP untill you fall asleep

If above does not help

- Go to the kitchen and have a very small snack.
- Back to the bed say slowly untill you fall asleep: sun, flower, seven, path, tee, run, yellow, apple, fish, rain, pen, water, smile, talk, life, sky.

If above does not help

- Say slowly untill morning: sun, flower, seven, path, tee, run, yellow, apple, fish, rain, pen, water, smile, talk, life, sky.

Day 7

Morning

* Whether you slept well or not, try to get out of bed between 6 and 7 o'clock. Never use an alarm clock. Your mind has a perfect feeling for the actual time, so rely on your mind and it will wake you up.

* Never be in a hurry.

* Repeat STOP to stop thinking.

* Say slowly to stop thinking : sun, flower, seven, path, tee, run, yellow, apple, fish, rain, pen, water, smile, talk, life, sky.

* Repeat slowly every hour: I do not care.

* Small physical excercise (20 min)

* Small breakfast.

* Nice talk (no complaints) 30 min. When nobody to talk with, phone or internet conversation oral or written.

* Walk 30 min.

* Imagine all the time people cannot wait to love you, but you must make the first step- a smile, a nice word or both. Only this! Do not be ashamed!

* Do not be serious with your own self. Be funny all the time or at least most of the time.

***

Afternoon

* Never be in a hurry.

* Repeat STOP (10 times every 30 hour)

* Say slowly every hour: sun, flower, seven, path, tee, run, yellow, apple, fish, rain, pen, water, smile, talk, life, sky.

* Repeat slowly every hour: I do not care.

* Dinner and half an hour break (you can sleep).

* Nice talk (no complaints) 30 min. When nobody to talk with, phone or internet conversation oral or written.

* Walk 30 min.

* Imagine all the time people cannot wait to love you, but you must make the first step- a smile, a nice word or both. Only this! Do not be ashamed!

* Do not be serious with your own self. Be funny all the time or at least most of the time.

***

Evening
- Never be in a hurry.
- Repeat STOP to stop thinking.
- Say slowly to stop thinking: sun, flower, seven, path, tee, run, yellow, apple, fish, rain, pen, water, smile, talk, life, sky.
- Repeat slowly every hour: I do not care.
- Small supper.
- Nice talk (no complaints) 30 min. When nobody to talk with, phone or internet conversation oral or written.
- Walk 30 min.
- Imagine all the time people cannot wait to love you, but you must make the first step- a smile, a nice word or both. Only this! Do not be ashamed!
- Do not be serious with your own self. Be funny all the time or at least most of the time.

***

Night
- Go to sleep before midnight (22.00- 24.00)

Before sleep
- Take a shower (warm water) 1 min.

- Small physical excercise 5 min.

In Bed

- ALWAYS ALONE during Sleeplessness Self Therapy.
- Repeat STOP to stop thinking.
- Say slowly untill you fall asleep: sun, flower, seven, path, tee, run, yellow, apple, fish, rain, pen, water, smile, talk, life, sky.
- Repeat slowly every hour: I do not care.

If you cannot fall asleep

- Say slowly untill you fall asleep: sun, flower, seven, path, tee, run, yellow, apple, fish, rain, pen, water, smile, talk, life, sky.

If above does not help

- Stand up and go to the toilet (when possible with as little light as possible)
- Say slowly untill you fall asleep: sun, flower, seven, path, tee, run, yellow, apple, fish, rain, pen, water, smile, talk, life, sky.

If above does not help

- Say STOP untill you fall asleep

If above does not help

- Go to the kitchen and have a very small snack.

- Back to the bed say slowly untill you fall asleep: sun, flower, seven, path, tee, run, yellow, apple, fish, rain, pen, water, smile, talk, life, sky.

If above does not help

- Say slowly untill morning: sun, flower, seven, path, tee, run, yellow, apple, fish, rain, pen, water, smile, talk, life, sky.

Congratulations! You made the Sleeplessness Self Therapy SST and you can finally sleep well. If after 14 days however this is not the case repeat the SST as long as necessary again and again.

P. W. Ariveder

www.ingramcontent.com/pod-product-compliance
Lightning Source LLC
Chambersburg PA
CBHW050309220526
45465CB00005B/1912